A Holistic Assessment Framework for Nurses

Cheryl Barnes-Neff, PhD, RN

Also by Cheryl Barnes-Neff

Compassion Centered C.A.R.E. series:

C.A.R.E. About What Matters Workshop
Compassion Centered C.A.R.E. Introduction
The Foundations of Compassion Centered C.A.R.E.
C.A.R.E. Notes

Open Hearted: Essays on Buddhist Study and Practice

Religion, Education, and Democracy: Exploring the Intersection between Religion, Secularism, Democracy, and Public Education in a Pluralistic America

A Holistic Assessment Framework for Nurses

PART OF THE
COMPASSION CENTERED C.A.R.E SERIES

Cheryl Barnes-Neff, PhD, RN

Laurel Oak Press

Laurel Oak Press is an imprint of Laurel Oak Group, LLC
by Cheryl Barnes-Neff. —1st ed.

Compassion Centered C.A.R.E.™ Series ISSN: 2771-1528
ISBN: 978-1-952017-05-6

Disclaimer: The information provided in this book is meant solely for informational and educational purposes only. The information contained here does not constitute legal, financial, medical, ethical, or professional advice. Always consult with your Country or State's regulatory statues, and your facility's policies and procedures to guide your care.

Important note: Any and all patient and staff related descriptions or stories have been modified to protect confidentiality and privacy. The essence of the stories is true.

Laurel Oak Group, LLC
P.O. Box 5295
Winter Park, FL 32793

Table of Contents

Love and compassion are
necessities, not luxuries.
Without them,
humanity cannot survive.
~ the Dalai Lama

CHAPTER 1

Why Compassion?

What is compassion, and why is it important in healthcare?

I've seen many patient care models come and go over my forty years as a nurse. From team nursing, to primary care, to care management, all the way to today's most popular model, patient centered care. Patient centered care is certainly a step in the right direction, and has many good points.

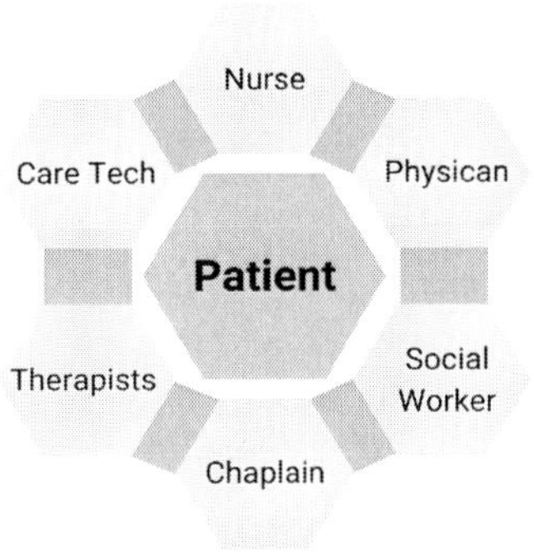

I'm proposing that our care model should actually be Compassion Centered C.A.R.E. When the patient is in the center of care, the model surrounds the patient with the different disciplines of healthcare professionals, but it implies that we're all doing something *to* the patient, not *with* the patient.

With compassion in the center, we're applying compassion to ourselves, our co-workers, and to our patients and their families. Work moves from being something that expects us to give and give without receiving, to a flow. The current model and systems are not sustainable, despite our herculean efforts to make it work. We exhaust ourselves for the sake of our patients, but it doesn't have to be that way. Work can also be part of a flow of giving and receiving that nourishes us as we nurture those around us.

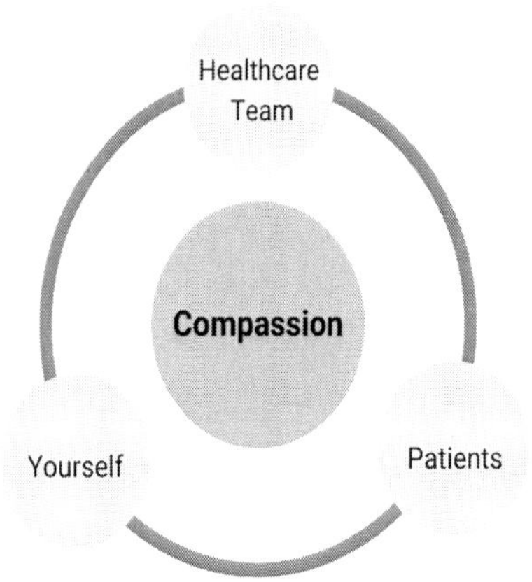

While I can't promise that the system will change overnight, I can say that as each of us embrace the idea that compassion can be centered, the model will move toward a more humane way of looking at the work that we do. We will all benefit. Our patients will feel heard and respected for who they are, our co-workers will understand that they are truly part of a team, and we will feel connected to our purpose of a life well lived.

What is Compassion?

There are a number of terms that are used somewhat interchangeably, and that can cause confusion. Words like pity, sympathy, empathy, caring, and compassion are used to describe our feelings when confronted with human suffering. I'd like to propose that we focus on two words: empathy and compassion.

Empathy is the feeling we get when we're touched emotionally by a fellow human who is suffering, and sometimes we not only feel badly that they are suffering, but we can also connect to a feeling within ourselves that resonates. We can never feel exactly the same way another person feels, but we can have a feeling of *Sympatico,* or a feeling of caring and mutual understanding with that person. The problem with empathy is that, while having a empathetic nature is part of what makes life wonderful, it can take us to the brink of empathic distress when we don't know what to do with that feeling.

Compassion includes feelings, but with the added dimension of the intention to act to ease the burden of suffering in the other person. Borrowing from the Buddhist tradition, that desire to act is seen as a response grounded in wisdom within an ethical framework.

What Problems Are We Trying To Solve?

A growing body of research is proving that compassion is more than just "nice to have" in healthcare professionals, it actually saves lives! Compassion is more than "the right thing to do." In the book *Compassionomics*, researchers Stephen Trzeciak and Anthony Mazzerelli spent two years combing through data, studies, and meta analyses discovering that the presence of compassion improved patient outcomes, and just as important, the lack of compassion had devastating consequences.

Does treating patients with compassion really matter?

The answer is far reaching. Compassion matters for patients physiologically, psychologically, socially, and spiritually; motivates self-care and compliance, improves healthcare quality, and improves an organization's bottom line. Oh, and it's an antidote to burnout.

Yet, with all of this goodness, there is a compassion crisis in healthcare. A literal crisis!

You may have read articles recently touting the goodness of compassion and empathy – there's hardly a magazine or website that talks about healthcare that hasn't published an article about empathy and compassion, and how we need more of them. Yet, there is pushback to this idea.

Some of the complaints about the call for more

compassion, empathy, and caring in healthcare include: "But, I just don't have time!" "If you care too much, it will break your heart and lead to burnout" and "It doesn't matter what the bedside manner is like, it's if the patient gets out alive that counts." And there's no denying that healthcare has many systemic problems that lead to real challenges in delivering care the way we want to. No one goes into nursing thinking that they will be cold and heartless to people in need, yet when we search our hearts, we've all had days that turned out like that. We make those excuses to keep those days from being more painful than we can bear.

What would it be like if you could come home after your shift – tired for sure – but satisfied that you were able to provide the compassionate care that you would want for your loved ones or for yourself? Care that every patient deserves.

I sincerely believe that staff do care, but sometimes they don't know the best way to provide compassionate care. What are some of the most common problems you're facing?

- ✓ Your staff are frustrated trying to create individualized patient plans of care.
- ✓ Satisfaction surveys coming back low on the "listened and showed respect for the patient" section. Studies show that when that question is answered positively, overall scores are higher.
- ✓ Staff are burned out, not engaged, bullying each other, and generally not happy.
- ✓ You know your staff care, but sometimes they don't know how to be compassionate.
- ✓ You're so frustrated, you're considering going back to the bedside, or leaving nursing all together.

You want your staff to care about each other and your patients. You've tried education and in-services, you may have even tried progressive discipline, or letting staff go to try to turn things around, and nothing seems to work.

The problem is that you've never had a step by stop process to use to teach your staff how to put compassion into action.

CHAPTER 2

Can Compassion Help?

I've made mistakes working with patients, and have gone home in tears because I couldn't give the care I wanted to give. I was told that I had to harden my heart to my patients' pain or I wouldn't make it. There were times that I took that advice, wanting to be an ICU badass: clinical all the way through. But then, a patient or a patient's family would pierce my heart with their pain – pain that came from the depth of their love.

Once, when I was waiting in the lobby for a friend that was having a minor procedure done, a surgeon came out to find a patient's family, calling "Loved ones! I'm looking for the loved ones of Mrs. Smith."

I just loved that! I started referring to my patient's "loved ones" ever since.

Compassion in healthcare has been part of my professional and personal journey throughout my life.

The Coronavirus crisis has brought the need for compassion into sharp relief. Personally, I think this is a watershed moment for all of us. On the site *"Dear World,"* nurses have been telling their stories of becoming more aware of the need for compassion than ever before. A nurse named Sarah Wells told her story of having the "hardened shell" around her heart broken. She explains about her patient:

"This day was her last and she was spoken to mostly through a glass door or by people garbed up - she didn't even know what her caregivers looked like. How terrifying. Losing a patient is never easy, but the nature of caring for trauma patients has a way of hardening you.

This day, the hardened shell I had built completely shattered and the tears were plentiful. Those around me commented, 'What's wrong with you? We do this every day!' I felt the same way, but I couldn't control it."[1]

My guess is that you've had a similar experience – I know I have. And on those days, we have an important choice to make. To allow that shell to be forever shattered, and bring compassion into all of our care, or to stay cocooned by pain.

For decades now, I've been working on the problem of what compassionate care looks like. Starting in the Neonatal Intensive Care Unit, and working my way to hospice as both a nurse and chaplain, I've trained new nurses, chaplains and social workers, and volunteers on how they can bring their compassion into the world.

---

[1] #DearNurses. *Dear World.org.* https://nurses.dearworld.org/013-I-ve-Never-Cried-Like-That-About-A-Patient-1

Lots of the suggestions you'll read if you do a search on "How is compassion shown in nursing?" will include things like making eye contact, treating the patient with kindness, holding their hand, and giving them your full attention. All of those things are good, but they don't go far enough.

I've developed a four-step process to be applied to yourself, your co-workers and staff, and to your patients and their families.

The C.A.R.E. Process

One of the hallmarks of compassionate care is often referred to as simply being the Golden Rule: Do unto others as you would have them do unto you. The problem comes in when we start working with the wide variety of patients and their families, and our co-workers. We live in a pluralistic society, and even in groups that seem to be pretty much the same, there is a wide array of opinions and preferences.

Better might be called the Platinum Rule: Treat

others the way they want to be treated. In other words, we have to ask them to know how they want to be treated. The C.A.R.E. process will lead you and your staff through finding out what is important to the patient through responding to them with dignity and respect, the heart of compassion.

Here's how it works: C.A.R.E. is an acronym for Connect, Assess, Respond, and Evaluate and End the encounter. These are steps you can implement right now to improve your life as a nurse leader, increase staff engagement and performance, and improve the satisfaction of your patients.

It's applied first to yourself. It's important that you understand the process on a personal level, and for you to exemplify the process to your staff and patients. This can't be a "do as I say, not as I do" kind of thing!

It's next applied to your staff and co-workers. Understanding your staff, and helping them understand each other will help in your efforts for improved communication, respectful behavior, and engagement and morale.

Finally, it's applied to your patients and their families. When the staff sees you listening to them, it's a light bulb effect, and they naturally take that ideal of listening to their patients. Let's look at each step.

Connect

Connection is what human beings need, thrive on, and long for. When we connect with others, we feel a sense of security, trust, being understood, and belonging. Connecting to ourselves might sound a bit strange at first, but the simple act of taking a breath – from the tip of our nose, to the tips of our toes – reconnects us to our bodies and is instantly refreshing.

Connecting to our staff helps to build team work, and helps them feel heard, and understood. Our patients, too, need that feeling of connection to feel safe. They come to us feeling uncertain, and even terrified. Simply making eye contact with a smile can be the beginning of building the trusting relationship they need on their path to recovery.

Assess

Assessment is what nurses do best, and we're going to take our assessment skills to the next level. When we assess our patients, we are really good at recognizing and understanding their bodily structures and functions. We use charting checklists that guide us through a head-to-toe systems review. What is sometimes missing are patient preferences, their social determinants of health, and the support they need. This sounds like a tall order, but it actually boils down to asking a single question: "What matters to you?"

There are many uses for this simple question, both to better understand our patients – to know who they are as people – as well as better understanding our staff and co-workers. When staff feel heard, they can express the underlying reasons for how they react to the things that upset them. When they feel heard, they feel more connected and part of a team.

When we assess ourselves, we not only ask ourselves "What matters to me?" but we can also take time to explore our assumptions about ourselves, our staff, and our patients. We need to ask "Is that true?" or "Am I sure?" and interrogate that assumption. We might find that when we get curious, when we start listening to their story, we make more room for empathy and compassion. One of my favorite quotes of Mr. Rogers is:

"Frankly, there isn't anyone you couldn't learn to love once you've heard their story."

Which leads to Respond

When we react to a situation, we often say or do things we later regret. We might feel the reaction is justified, but when we look back, we have that feeling that we wish we had done things differently. I've been there – more than once.

But we can learn to respond instead of react. Let's add "respond with respect" to the mix as well. When we know the person's story, we still might not agree with their choices or decisions, but we do get a little closer to understanding why they are the way they are. We get to know them as person.

When we do that, we can get a lot closer to giving them the best possible care. Remember our analogy above about the Platinum Rule? The people we care for are unique individuals, so when it comes time to provide care, communicate with them, or connect with them, it needs to be on their terms. Then the compassionate action becomes action that will actually serve them; not just a canned checkmark on a list of interventions.

This becomes the individualized plan of care. A discharge plan the patient can actually follow.

Did a lightbulb just go off? I know, right?

Evaluate and End the Encounter

No nursing process would be complete without spending a moment on evaluating the interaction. Did our interventions work? We can also add looking at how well we were able to connect with our patients, were we able to assess their situation honestly, and respond to them with compassion?

Applying this to ourselves and our staff is also important. Having an end of shift checklist for ourselves can be enlightening and helpful. Not as a way to beat ourselves up, but to look at the progress we're making, and if this method is working.

In Joan Halifax's book *Standing at the Edge*, she offers sage advice for engaging with the suffering we see all around us with integrity. While I've developed and used my C.A.R.E. model over the past decades of work, I was inspired by Roshi Joan's addition of *End* to the process. She says, "When the time is right, we mark the end of our time… so that we can move cleanly to the next moment, person, or task." She goes on to say, "Without the acknowledgment of what has taken place, it can be difficult to let go of this encounter and move on." This is so important.

Have you ever found that you wake up at 3 in the morning worrying (or is it just me?), or that you spend time worrying about work when you're home, only to turn around and worry about home while you're at work?

Having a definitive *End* to our interactions and encounters goes a long way to solve this problem, bring peace of mind to our lives.

I've been working in the hospice field for the past twenty years, and one of the things I learned early on was to say goodbye to my patients at the end of every visit. Even if it was just to make eye contact, and hold their hand with a smile. The reality is that we might not see that patient again.

We might have a little ritual of being sure we at least wave bye to each of our staff at the end of the shift, touch base with anyone who needs help to finish, and to have our own "goodbye" before leaving the floor. Even something as simple as taking off our lanyard, hanging it in our locker, and saying "see you tomorrow."

CHAPTER 3

C.A.R.E. for Our Patients

C.A.R.E. for Our Patients

Let's take a look at the steps of C.A.R.E. applied to patient care. The process allows us to recognize our patients as individuals with their own priorities, preferences, and choices.

Connect

Connections matter. When we have human connection, we feel a sense of security, trust, being understood, and belonging. Connect with your patients by establishing rapport. Call them by their preferred name, pronouns, et cetera. Connecting with patients is a crucial part of the patient's feeling of confidence that they will be cared for. They're often frightened and anxious about what is happening, and may feel no one truly cares about them. Everything we do and say makes an impact on them. So we must be careful not to cause them more anxiety and concern.

To make a connection, we can make eye contact, shake hands if appropriate, and make sure we call them by the correct name, pronouns, and have a caring stance.

In some cultures, being smiley and cheerful when they are sick and worried might seem insensitive. A smile and a fleeting touch can telegraph a feeling of care, and studies show that "grammy-grandpa" talk harms patients. You've probably heard staff talk with an elder in that kind of, "How are we doing today, Pops?" or, "Oh, you're so cute!" as they pat the patient on the head. Patients with dementia are less cooperative and more combative when spoken to as though they are children. Instead, call each patient by the name may prefer. For some, that name may be a different than the one that's on their medical record. We want to be sure to balance patient safety for identification, treatments, and medication administration, while honoring the patient's priorities around their name and identity.

For elders, it's best to call them by their surname and last name. They may say it's okay to call them by a nickname, but until you've known them for awhile, err on the side of honor and respect.

Be sure to remember consent. Ask permission to touch, and be sure to describe what's going on in detail, and what will be done to the patient step-by-step. Understand cultural aspects of personal contact, and have cultural humility. Don't assume you know, be sure to ask.

Assess

Assess your patient and their family. In addition to head to toe assessment ask: "What matters to you?" Listen to the answers, learn what their healthcare priorities are, and learn about their culture, family dynamics, and home life. The answers are the basis of what we should do for them.

To understand our patients, we need to know who they are as people. We want to know what is wrong with the patient and what concerns have brought to them to us for care, of course, but we also want to know what matters to them as people. We can ask a number of questions to find out more about their priorities, what social determinants of health are present that might affect their care, and what their support needs are. It's important to know what family, culture, religion, social situation, and other aspects might impact their life. We might find that when we get curious, when we start listening to their story, we make more room for empathy and compassion.

Listening Skills

We like to think of ourselves as good listeners, but it's important to take a closer look at our listening skills. Listening is a key component of assessment.

We need to discover the patient's history, their chief complaints, and their observations and reports about their symptoms. There are a number of types of listening, and it's important to be able to identify them. We might: not be listening, we might listen from habit, listen to form a response, listen with an open mind, listen with an open heart, and listen with compassion - being fully present.

Not Listening

Sometimes we have to admit we're not actually listening at all. We may think that we can look at the phone, answer emails, check the news, look at social media posts all the while carrying on a conversation. But the reality is, we really can't do all of that at the same time. Our modern life has created an erosion of our attention spans – some reports even claim that we have attention spans shorter than a goldfish!

And we have the pressure of marketers competing for our attention. In a sense, our attention is the commodity that they most covet. Recapturing our attention, and learning to not be so easily distracted for ourselves would add to our quality of life.

Listening Out of Habit

Sometimes we listen out of habit. Maybe we think we've heard the same thing so many times, we know what comes next. Maybe we're mind reading since we don't really trust that they know what they're saying, and we're going to correct their narrative. We are being disrespectful when we do this.

You may have seen some of the videos on social media of nurse influencers who tease and mock the various types of nurses giving report: the confused one, the disorganized one, the too many details one, the not enough detail one, and so on. Anytime we think we can pigeon hole someone, we risk listening out of habit. This can trip us up when something new is added, or we're caught not really listening.

Listening to Form an Argument

We may have been guilty of listening in order to form an argument or other response. We're assuming that we know what they're going to say. We know we disagree, so we want to be ready with a clever retort. Or, we can't wait to share our similar experience with them, defeating their desire to share their feeling or experience with us, only to have us say, "Oh, I know exactly how you feel. That happened to me, too!"

Listening With an Open Mind

Other ways to listen, include listening with an open mind – we're willing to learn. We take in new information, asking questions to clarify and note differences. During a patient assessment, this quality is especially important. We may find that sometimes the way a patient describes their symptoms doesn't match the way we in the medical field would. You may have had a patient who denies that they have any pain, yet you can see them guarding the injured part, or grimacing when they're moved or touched. When we ask what it feels like, they may describe a "deep ache," or "like a hot poker," or "pins and needles." They don't consider it "pain," yet they do need pain management for their somatic, neurologic, or visceral pain.

Listen With an Open Heart

We can also listen with an open heart. We can see through the other person's eyes, making an emotional connection. We set aside our personal point of view for a moment in order to understand that, while their response to a situation might be different from ours, it is their truth. Our open heart helps us to recognize their feelings, and to be able to process and restate our understanding of their feelings.

Listening With Compassion

Listening with compassion means that we're fully present with the other person. We're calm and have the stability needed to be with them, even when they're in a lot of pain; even when we're feeling uncomfortable. An old habit might be to try to fix. As Brené Brown mentioned in her presentation, putting a silver lining around their pain. When that happens, it's important to take a breath, reconnect with ourselves, and recognize what's happening within us. Then we can return to listening and being present with the patient. We're willing not to have the answers or try to fix the problem, but we're partnering with them to companion them on their journey.

Respond

We want to respond instead of react. Responding with respect, being sensitive to their cues, understanding the whole person, knowing the person's priorities of care, and deciding how to best approach the situation is the goal. Every human being deserves to be treated with dignity and respect. We want that for ourselves and our patients want that as well.

Following the patient's cues is important. You've probably heard the phrase, the "COPD personality" (often said with an eye roll), but why are COPD patients sometimes impatient. They often have to manage their energy very carefully. If they get out of breath before a meal, they may not be able to eat their full meal because of being out of breath. So if you go into the room before mealtime and ask them a bunch of questions, they may very well tell you to get lost. Not being able to breathe is terrifying and they want to avoid a crisis above all else.

In order to follow our Platinum Rule, we need to understand the whole person. Each of us is more than the sum of our parts. When we take a look at their values, culture, religious practices, and family dynamics, we get a better picture of who they are as a person. Knowing the patient's priorities of care, allows us to better plan their care and discover the social determinants of health affecting them.

When we understand that, we realize that if their choices are different from ours, that's okay. We can let ourselves off the hook. They don't have to follow what we say. In fact, we're far more likely to find a solution that they can follow, when we know those priorities and preferences.

Understanding where the patient is coming from and what issues impact them, can help us respond to their needs, and sometimes demands, appropriately when we've connected first with ourselves, and then with them as an individual. Our response is a decision that will help them.

There will be times when responding with respect will be challenging. We've all had experiences with patients who were disrespectful or even combative with us. It's tough to keep that from affecting how we react to them. Taking the high road can feel less than gratifying, but in the long run, keeping our cool and living up to our values of being respectful and compassionate is worth it.

Evaluate and End

Lastly, we Evaluate and End the encounter with the

patient. Were the interventions you planned effective? Did you gain the bigger picture of the patient's life? Is the plan of care individualized in a real way, and did the patient understand and have confidence in the plan? When thinking about the plan of care for the patient, does it reflect their priorities, support needs, and limitations? Will they be able to comply with the discharge plan or is the plan just wishful thinking? Do they understand what's happening? And does it make sense to them in their worldview?

Take a moment after the interaction with the patient to consider not only the medical evaluation, but your personal one as well. Were you able to use the C.A.R.E. process effectively? How did it go? Did you gain a bigger picture of the person's life? Do you feel you connected with them in a meaningful way? Did you empathize with them, even if you've never experienced what they're going through, or even if you disagree with their reactions and decisions?

When ending an interaction with a patient, leave that interaction peacefully. Even if things didn't go as well as you'd hoped, understand that all of this takes practice and there will be times that even the very best of plans and intentions won't be successful.

You may also leave with a sense that you really did connect with the patient and have a clearer understanding of them. That's something to celebrate! Wish them well and move on to the next task, giving that next interaction your full attention.

CHAPTER 6

Holistic Assessment

An important part of Compassion Centered C.A.R.E. is expanding our knowledge of nursing assessment to include a holistic approach to care. In this context, holistic refers to the understanding that each of us is more than the sum of our parts. We learn in nursing school about the medical aspects of care, but sometimes other factors that impact care like psychosocial needs, cultural considerations, and the many social determinants of health are not emphasized. These factors are crucial if we are to provide compassionate care that is centered on the needs and priorities of the patient, and that look critically and realistically at the patient's reality and their world view.

I'll introduce a simple framework of doing a holistic assessment that will work for you regardless of your organization's charting system. And, we'll see how this framework will make your care and discharge plans more effective. The goal is always to help our patients by easing the burden of their suffering, and partnering with them for the best possible long term care and support. You'll find that this framework is also very satisfying for you as a nurse or other healthcare professional. By listening to our patients in an objective and nonjudgmental way, we can release the stress we sometimes feel when we believe we must give the patient the one right plan, and if that plan isn't followed, we've somehow failed. By creatively and open-heartedly, trusting our patients to know what's best for them at any given time, we treat them with respect and they feel that they can trust us. Listening builds trust, and trust builds confidence in accepting and taking our best advice. Especially, when that advice takes their needs and values into account.

More Than the Sum of Our Parts

Each person we meet is more than the sum of their parts, yet when learning about healthcare, in order to break down the enormous amount of information we need to learn, we break this knowledge down into its component parts. Any person coming to us for healthcare, has a medical condition and its associated problem list. We need to do a head to toe assessment, often breaking down the assessment into the major systems of the body. We look at the body's structure and function, but sometimes forget to incorporate the other aspects of what it means to be a human being.

Additionally, we need to bear in mind that the patient's psychosocial, spiritual, cultural, attitudes about healthcare including their past interactions with healthcare professionals and organizations, other beliefs, and how the patient wants and needs to be communicated with, affects the assessment. While we won't be the expert at all of these dimensions, it's important that we are aware of them and how they impact the patient's current condition, what their plan of care needs to include, and how to create a successful discharge plan for the patient. We also want to be aware of any risk factors that necessitate a referral to the appropriate professional in that role. Social Workers, Counselors, Board Certified Chaplains, Child Life Specialists, Therapists, and others, will be able to assist the patient and their family within their scope of practice. Don't forget to double back and review their findings. It 's important to have the full picture in mind to assure the best possible care for our patients, and the most successful discharge plan.

This graph illustrates a fuller picture of the patient. Understanding that the medical aspect of their lives are not necessarily the most dominant concern. Because we devote our lives to learning and dealing with medical conditions, we have a bias toward putting medical care first. Often patients prioritize other aspects of their lives over the medical or "taking care of themselves." The goal for healthcare really isn't "compliance," even though we have a hard time letting that idea go. Our goal is actually to help find the plan of care that includes all aspects of the patient's world view, promotes trust in the healthcare professionals on their team, and enhances communication between all these individuals.

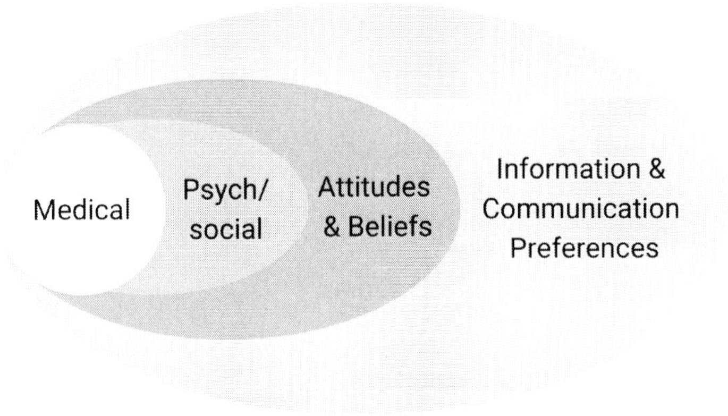

International Classification of Functioning, Disability, and Health

The World Health Organization has created an International Classification of Functioning, Disability, and Health – also known as the ICF. The ICF is an important innovation in the way we look at disability. It standardizes the characterization of structural and functional impairments, and relates them to a patient's activity limitations and participation restrictions. It goes further by looking closely at the support a patient needs, and correlates those needs with the resources available within the context of their environment and world view.

Components of the ICF:

- ❖ Functioning and disability
  - ✓ Body functions and structures
  - ✓ Includes psychosocial, emotional, mental illness, and family dynamics
  - ✓ Activities and participation
- ❖ Contextual Factors
  - ✓ Environmental factors
  - ✓ Personal factors

This grid illustrates the dimensions of a health condition, connecting the factors involved. You can see that this grid places "activities" at the center of the patient's health condition. This helps us see that disability is actually a continuum and where the patient falls on that continuum can change, and will certainly be affected by the levels of support available to them.

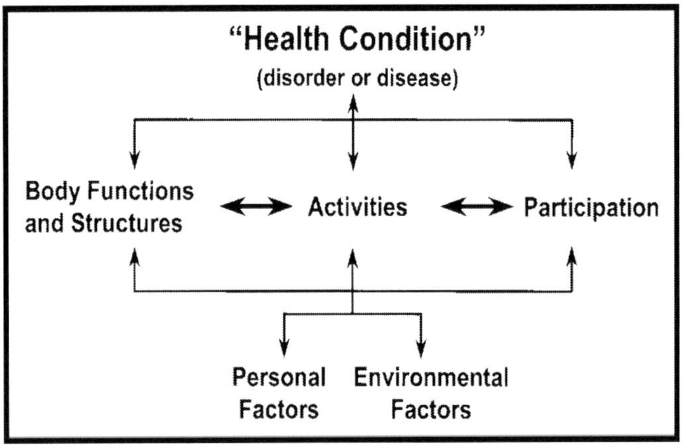

The contextual factors involved in the patient's support include environmental factors made up of the physical, social, emotional, and cultural world of the patient. These contextual factors include:

products and technology, support and relationships, attitudes and culture, services systems and policies.

- Environmental factors make up the physical, social, emotional, and cultural world of the patient
    - Products and technology
    - Support and relationships
    - Attitudes and culture
    - Services, systems, and policies

It is a sad fact of life that not all people have the same access to support for their medical needs. It's important for each of us to not only be aware of these healthcare inequities, but to look for ways to even the playing field for our patients. Systemic racism, sexism, ageism, and ableism can seem invisible to those of us unaffected by these systemic inequities.

We need to make a commitment to ourselves to educate ourselves on these issues, and to interrogate our assumptions about our patients, and understand what hurdles they must overcome. By understanding these issues, listening to and believing our patients when they express their frustrations with these problems, and not being afraid to recognize our role in these systems is crucial.

Keeping an open mind, and keeping an eagle eye out for these issues can help us be proactive in helping our patients overcoming these hurdles. We want to be part of the solution for our patients, not part of the problem!

CHAPTER 7

The Basics of Assessment

Structure and function is the most common approach to assessment. We're all familiar with the assessment checklist that focuses on structure, function, and symptoms. For the most part, this part of the assessment is easy and straightforward. We can use our four senses to assess: touch and palpation, listening to heart and other internal sounds, observing the external structures and movement, and even smell in the case of wound infections. We use diagnostic methods to assess the patient's systems and function. X-rays and scans, lab results, monitoring, and other methods enhance and confirm our assessments.

Structure and Function

- Is the structure sound?
- Does everything function?
- Are there structural impairments?
- Are there functional limitations?
- What are the patient's symptoms?

Becoming not only competent but expert at assessment is a major goal for all healthcare professionals. Then it's important to broaden our horizons to include all of the dimensions of a person and their world view.

Impairments

- Problems in body function or structure such as significant deviation or loss:
    - ✓ Mental functions
    - ✓ Sensory functions and pain
    - ✓ Functions of body systems

Once we assess and understand the patient's problems with the structure and function of their bodily systems, the next step is to understand the limitations these problems place on the patient. The patient will be affected by the patient's mental functions, their sensory functions and pain, and the functions of their body systems.

Many factors enter into the patient's perception of their health problems. A patient who has been lucky and has never been ill or had a major injury before, may be quite shocked at their condition. They may have been less than empathetic with others who have illness or injury because they had no frame of reference; it's hard to believe that this "hurts so much!" or they may become very worried or even obsessed with what will happen next. "How could this happen to me?" might be something you'll hear these kinds of patients say. Patients who have been "health nuts" and feel they did everything right, may feel that their medical problem can't be true.

On the other hand, you may have patients who

have had chronic illnesses or disabilities for a long time; even for most of their lives. They may feel that they have had to fight with the healthcare system to get what they need. They've heard all the questions, and can be quite weary of hearing the same questions – sometimes multiple times a day! They can also feel that healthcare professionals are judging or even blaming them for their condition. Mainly, they don't understand why we don't listen to them.

Subjective Symptoms

Pain and other symptoms are affected by these factors as well. Something that is very important to understand is that pain or other symptom scales are simply a way for the patient to compare their perception of pain or other symptoms. Pain is always subjective. The pain scale does not turn a subjective experience into an objective observation. It's important to recognize that the pain score is NOT a dosing guide. When a pain naïve patient reports that their pain is on the severe end of the scale, that report does not mean that we abandon good pain management principles. We still "start low and go slow," and have close and consistent evaluation of the patient's pain. A patient who has had chronic pain for years might report their pain at 4 with a goal of 2, but the medication type and dosage might be what we'd expect only for someone in severe pain. The reality is that, if we could experience that patient's pain, we'd probably be knocked to our knees!

Also important to realize that a patient's perception of their pain is strongly affected by their emotional state. If they feel very emotional, perhaps they are going through a personal trauma like a divorce, or being estranged from their family, or feeling spiritual despair, they may report their pain being very intense. Again, we start low and go slow with their pain medication, but when there are emotional, spiritual, or psychological issues compounding the situation, we won't be able to get their pain under control without addressing these issues. A consult with the Social Worker, Licensed Mental Health Counselor, or Board Certified Chaplain may go a long way in helping the patient.

Another patient might feel that they're being a burden on us, or that they are weak if they admit that they have pain. We need to observe if they are guarding the part that is affected, their facial expression, tone of voice, ability to ambulate, appetite, quality of sleep, and others clues that show that they are experiencing pain. Helping them to voice their concerns, perhaps bringing in the Social Worker to ask the "why" question, can help in understanding and working with the underlying problems to find a way to palliate the patient's pain. This will enhance the patient's over-all wellness and quality of life.

The most important thing to remember is that we must use our professional knowledge of care and treatment, and to include the complexities of how our patients perceive their condition. Just because we've observed a procedure many times, and might even believe that it doesn't really hurt that much, or it's really not a big deal, that doesn't mean that the patient has that kind of confidence in what's happening to them. They can be terrified by what we consider routine.

Activity Limitations

Limitations are what is most important to our patients. When a patient has physical structural, functional, or symptom problems, the limitations this places on the patient's life is at the forefront of the patient's mind.

Limitations

- Activity limitations
- Participation restrictions
    - ✓ Mobility
    - ✓ Self-care
    - ✓ Relationships and interactions
    - ✓ Community and social life

A simple example would be a patient who has a broken arm. If the left arm is broken, and the patient is right handed, the limitation is less than if the dominant arm is affected. You can probably think of more examples along this line. Someone who works in an office environment, may be able to use a voice activated system on their computer so they can continue their work with only minor inconvenience. On the other hand, if a construction worker breaks their arm, they may be out of work for weeks as the break heals. Or, they may choose to continue to work, but be really hard on the cast, and not follow the recommendations for limiting the range of motion in the associated joints.

All of us have important activities that we need to continue to stay healthy and survive, and to enjoy our lives. Mobility and self-care are important for all of us. For our patients, limitations on their basic activities of daily living and self-care can be factors that either allow the patient to recover, or that will lead to decline in the patient's condition, maybe even creating a life limiting situation.

Part of what makes life worth living is our ability

to interact with others and create healthy relationships. We thrive when we have these individual relationships, and can interact with our community, and have an active social life. When these relationships are limited, our health can suffer even further.

This chart gives an example of a scale that could be used to evaluate a patient's limitations. When we can measure the patient's limitations based on their individual circumstances, we can look at ways we can support them. We can also use a chart like this to evaluate the plan of care and treatments provided. There will be situations when the patient's limitations won't be possible to improve due to their disability. However, this does not mean that we have no further care to provide. We continue to be creative in looking for ways to mitigate the patient's perceptions of their limitations, ways to bring other aspects of their life to the forefront, and how to use technology, durable medical equipment, or social support to meet the patient's needs.

Level	Description	Qualifiers
0	None	No limitations
1	Mild	Present < 25% of the time, tolerable, happen rarely over the last 30 days
2	Moderate	Present < 50% of the time, interfering with day to day life, happens occasionally over the last 30 days
3	Severe	Present > 50% of the time, partially disrupting day to day life, happens frequently over the last 30 days
4	Complete	Present > 95% of the time, totally disrupting day to day life, happens every day over the last 30 days

For example, a young man who had progressive muscular degeneration felt socially isolated and very lonely. By providing him with a laptop computer, he was able to enter a community college system and take online classes that included real time class discussions. There were online social games and forums he participated in with good success.

While it wasn't possible for him to travel often, he was able to be transported to the college for the end of his favorite class using an electric wheelchair to attend with his classmates and connect in person. Appropriate support made all the difference.

Contextual Factors

I'm sure the role of contextual factors in the patient's condition is becoming clear. When a patient is in our environment, we can forget that the limitations in their environment can have a big impact.

Contextual Factors

- Environmental factors make up the physical, social, emotional, and cultural world of the patient
    - Products and technology
    - Support and relationships
    - Attitudes and culture
    - Services, systems, and policies

The patient's environmental factors make up the

physical, social, emotional, and cultural world of the patient can include: products and technology, support and relationships, attitudes and culture, and services, systems, and policies. We looked at the over-view of these points, so let's look at a few examples of how these might affect individual patients.

We mentioned the young man who was able to utilize a computer with network capabilities and a motorized wheelchair to enhance his quality of life, and there are many more examples. The patient's family, community, religion, culture, and other societal factors can make a big difference in a patient's condition, progress, and healing efforts. When a patient's plan of care includes medications that are not part of their insurance policy's formulary, and the patient cannot afford the medication, they will not be able to take that medication. Rather than judging them "non-compliant," we can look closer to find other medications or provide help in appealing insurance company decisions. For patients without insurance, this becomes even more important and challenging for the team to respond to.

World View

The patient's family, culture, religious, and social rules and norms can make a big difference as well. A patient may believe in the cultural remedies of their family and ancestors. They may value these remedies more than the medical care we recommend. They might even hide their desire to use these traditions if they feel we will be judgmental or forbid them. By being open to their beliefs, we can assure that our plan of care accommodates these remedies, assuring there are no adverse interactions, or looking at the timing of medications and procedures. This will assure that the patient retains the support of their family and community, and illustrates our respect for dignity in their identity.

On the other hand, the patient's identity may be in conflict with their family and culture or religion. For example, a transgender patient may be rejected by their family and be considered as going against strongly held religious beliefs. They may find themselves homeless or searching for a sympathetic community for support. When working with this patient, sensitivity is important. We need to assure that we use their preferred name and pronouns, and that we give extra care during a physical exam for privacy and consent. You may have noticed the use of "they" and "their" in the singular in this book. While that is not a common usage for many, it is correct and helps in emphasizing inclusion. In fact, in some organizations, it is common to see all staff's preferred pronouns on their name badge. This helps normalize asking for and using this information appropriately.

Patients might be part of a culture where the gendered rules are very strict for who makes decisions about the healthcare of the members of a family. The head of the household, often the elder male of the family might insist on making final decisions about care, medication, or other treatments. He might even dictate what can and cannot be shared with the patient about their condition. This can be common in end of life cases, and hospices often find families who want to shield their loved ones from the reality of their prognosis. Each healthcare professional must come to terms with these situations, which can fly in the face of our modern sensibilities about informed consent, veracity, and decision making. It can be difficult, but it is important to approach these situations with an open mind, looking for alternatives that will satisfy the root cause of the patients needs.

Peace of Mind

Even when a patient's culture goes against our strongly held beliefs, we must make an effort to interrogate our beliefs to find a way to accept the patient and their family in a way that is respectful of their dignity. We don't have to agree or join practices that we disagree with, but as long as it is not harming the patient, they have the right to their beliefs and practices. Our job is to support them in the best way we can. We can develop a sense of calmness and composure – equanimity – that will give us peace of mind.

Quality of Life

This chart, from the Centers for Disease Control and Prevention provides additional clarity on how the contextual factors affect the patient's disease progression as well as the place of contextual factors in the hierarchy of healthcare.

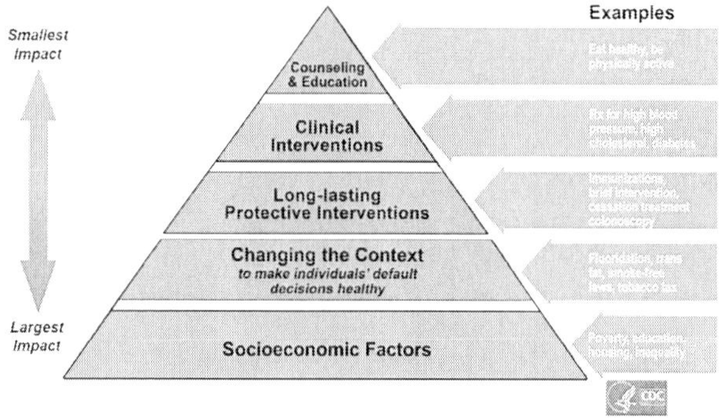

Adapted from Thomas R. Frieden. A Framework for Public Health Action: The Health Impact Pyramid. American Journal of Public Health: April 2010, Vol. 100, No. 4, pp. 590-595. doi: 10.2105/AJPH.2009.185652

You'll see that the socioeconomic factors are considered as having the largest impact on factors that affect health. We often think of our lifestyle choices to be the most important drivers in health, but this just isn't the case. While lifestyle can certainly help with quality of life, and there are risk factors involved, those factors are far less impactful than the patient's socioeconomic factors, systemic issues, equity disparity, and availability of protective interventions.

We'd love to believe that if we can just do everything right with our health, we'll be spared unpleasant conditions and diseases. You may have heard people say that if they eat a vegan diet, never smoke, or keep to a special (often expensive) diet or supplements, etc., they will be bullet-proof and never get sick. The reality is that patients who have never smoked or even been around smokers can develop lung cancer, and there are smokers who never develop respiratory illness. The fact of the matter is that many of these diseases are too complex to be able to chalk up to lifestyle choices that contribute less to the outcome than we might think.

Of course we want to encourage our patients to develop good habits and lifestyle choices that will enhance their quality of life. But we do need to be cautious that we don't wind up shaming our patients or blaming them for their condition.

Support

Support and connection are crucial for patients to heal and thrive. When a patient has limitations, finding and cultivating interpersonal support is so important. This support includes: self-care, relationships and interactions, community and social life, mobility, and financial support.

Support Factors

- What support is needed for the patient's limitations?
  - ✓ Self-care
  - ✓ Relationships & interactions
  - ✓ Community & social life
  - ✓ Mobility
  - ✓ Financial

Self-care can include things like finding time to do something fun or special like going to a movie or out to dinner, to the more in-depth care like prayer life and philosophical contemplation. In our relationships, we need connections with people who we can trust to have conversations with that share our inner most thoughts, fears, and concerns. These relationships can vary depending on the history between the individuals. In each of these, forming and maintaining healthy boundaries is a key area that will protect the relationships and the patient's well-being.

Community and social life is important to some patients. A person who is used to being involved in social, cultural, or religious groups, perhaps even being a leader in the organization may feel real grief when these activities are curtailed due to illness. As illness progresses, the role of the patient will shift and change in the family or social settings.

A man who has been the head of household, perhaps a leader in his work or community, may grieve the loss of his role when others in the family need to step in and take charge in many situations. In a family where mom has always taken care of everyone in the family, and has always been the one who always brings the best casserole to the pot luck, may find that members of the family and group are at a loss for how to care for her.

In any of these cases, it's important that we identify potential problems and work with the family to find solutions that may include bringing in outside caregivers, training for the family or friends, or other ways the patient's needs can be met within the context of the family situation.

CHAPTER 8

The Next Level

We can take assessment to the next level by recognizing that our observations need to include the factors that personalize the patient's priorities and life. When we assess any patient, when we've determined their structure and function, it's important to then ask questions about their limitations. Some of the questions we need to ask include:

- ✓ How does the patient respond to their limitations?
- ✓ How do they respond to the treatment for their problem?
- ✓ Are they being optimally treated?
- ✓ What resources are available to the patients?

Assessment Framework

Inspired by the WHO's ICF, this is a framework for assessment that includes the holistic factors that see the patient as a full person. Whether in the physical, psychosocial, or spiritual/cultural dimensions, we can assess by going through each aspect of the patient: structure, function, limitations, and support. Let's go through an example for physical problems first.

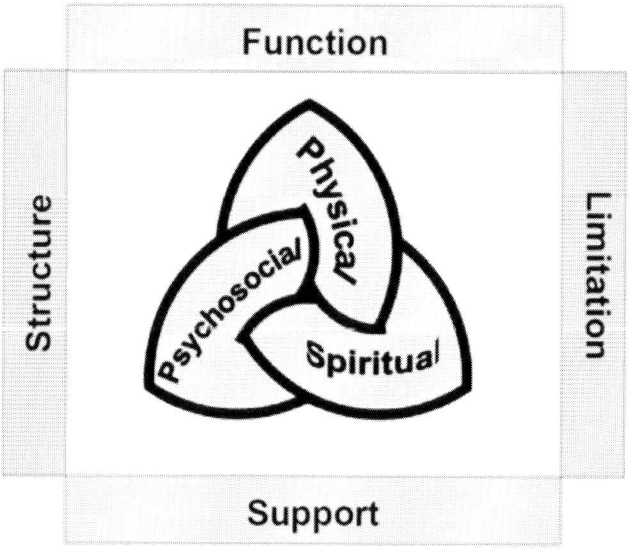

Structure

In looking at the patient's physical structure, we do a head-to-toe assessment using basic anatomy and physical systems. We may use a charting checklist to guide us.

Physical Structure:

- ✓ Head-to-Toe assessment
- ✓ Basic anatomy
- ✓ Physical systems
- ✓ Charting checklists

Function

Function is sometimes difficult to distinguish from the physical structure, and sometimes they are blended on your charting checklist. But think of function in terms of what the physical structure does in the body. Among these functions will be mobility issues, the pathophysiology of the disease process, and is measured with diagnostic test results, vital signs, and patient reported symptoms. Be sure to compare any of these results and measures over time. A single number isn't as meaningful to understanding the patient's condition as a continuum of their symptoms and other measures.

Physical Function:

- ✓ Mobility issues
- ✓ Pathophysiology
- ✓ Diagnostic test results
- ✓ Vital signs
- ✓ Compare results over time

Limitations

Understanding the limitations a condition has on a patient is key to developing an individualized plan of care. We discussed some possible scenarios where limitations can be a strong factor for the patient. During the assessment and throughout the patient's stay, an ongoing assessment will help your understanding of the patient's world view.

Be sure to ask about their symptoms, mobility issues, systemic limitations, and their understanding of their role or employment, the emotional impact of their illness, and their quality of life.

Physical Limitations:

- ✓ Symptoms
- ✓ Mobility issues
- ✓ Systemic limitations
- ✓ Patient reporting:
    - Role or employment
    - Emotional impact
    - Quality of life

Support

By looking at the support the patient needs, a discharge plan can be developed that will have a far greater chance of success for the patient than creating a plan that is a cookie cutter approach. When we take all of these factors into consideration, the patient will feel heard, and will be an active participant in their on-going healthcare.

Don't make assumptions – review with the patient what resources they have, and what they will need. This is an important time to take an interdisciplinary approach. If the case is complicated, the facility social worker will be able to make community connections for the patient to help with financial, social, and referral needs.

Physical Support:

- ✓ What support do they have?
- ✓ What support do they need?
  - Financial
  - Healthcare availability
  - Family help
  - Assistive devices
  - Medication

Patients do not respond as well when they have treatment plans dictated to them. In a holistic, patient-centered approach, the patient is an active participant in their care. We need to listen to what matters to them, what aspects affect the plan of care, and how the team can work together to come up with creative solutions that will be successful.

Nothing about me, without me

Dimensions of Life

We reviewed using the holistic assessment framework for the physical assessment, now let's take a look at using it with other dimensions of the patient's life. In the psychosocial dimension of the patient, we can look at a variety of aspects. Their emotional life, social and community life, and their relationship within their family unit.

Family Structure

When assessing the family, start with the structure

of the family. Find out who the members of the family are, and if anyone is missing. Remember that not all families have a traditional structure: they may have a blended family, be in a homosexual relationship, or have other configurations of members. A family tree, or genome, can be used to identify the members of a family, including their extended family. A genogram may be valuable to develop, and you may want to include the Social Worker or Board Certified Chaplain to help in it's development, especially if there is a complicated or particularly problematic family dynamic.

Family Structure:

- ✓ Who are they?
- ✓ Family tree
- ✓ Is anyone "missing?"
- ✓ Do they feel complete?

Family Function

The function of the members of the family, and the family as a whole unit are varied and complex. A major aspect to consider are the roles of the members of the family. It is very important for the healthcare professional to be nonjudgmental about the family structure and the roles within the family. If the family is unconventional, don't assume that it is dysfunctional. Look at the functions of the family members as objectively as possible.

We want to assess the roles of the family members, their identity as a family, or their place in society or cultural milieu. What are the responsibilities of the family members? This may play an important role if one of the members cannot fulfil their role, and another member must step in. Families often have expectations of each other, or their social circle or culture may have expectations of them to continue being considered part of the group.

Family Function:

- ✓ What are their roles?
- ✓ What is their identity as a family?
- ✓ Responsibilities?
- ✓ Expectations?

Limitations of the Family

Look at the limitations present in the family structure, if any. For some patients, especially those with chronic disabilities, there may be tensions in the family, both with caregiver fatigue, and with issues around the ongoing care of the patient. For example, an older man with chronic COPD who still smokes, may find that his wife is very resentful that he is not taking care of himself in her eyes. She may resist fully participating in his care, or forbid that he smoke again. This might lead him to hide his smoking, putting himself and his family at risk of fire if he smokes without turning off his oxygen concentrator.

Understanding the various factors is important. What is causing friction among family members? What problems are they experiencing? Are there other difficulties that will make caring for the patient difficult? And what are their needs? Often the family issues are a greater problem for patient discharge planning than the patient themselves.

Family Limitations:

- ✓ What factors cause limitations?
- ✓ Friction?
- ✓ Problems?
- ✓ Other difficulties?
- ✓ What are their needs?

Family Support

The patient's immediate family is an important source of support and help, but be sure to look past the immediate family to their extended family unit, friends, social community, faith community, etc. The patient may have access to additional resources, such as online support groups, searching for additional or alternative treatments, as well as organizations specializing in their condition.

Looking at the support they have, what their over-all needs are, and look for ways to fill the gaps so that the discharge plan has the best chance of on-going success.

Family Support:

- ✓ Other family?
- ✓ Social structure?
- ✓ Faith community?
- ✓ Financial?
- ✓ Technological?
- ✓ Access to resources?

Dimensions of Life

Each person has a variety of dimensions that are worthy of being assessed. The more complete our holistic assessment is, the better chance we have for success in developing a healthcare plan that they can live with. By understanding how these aspects work together and how interconnected they are, we will have a far more complete picture of the patient. We come into the patient interaction as the "content expert," but the patient is the "life expert."

We need to give our patients our best advice, knowledge about their condition, and information about treatment options. We are an important part of the team, but we are only one member of the team. The patient must be the team leader, so that they can live their best life. We need to have patience with this approach, because the patient's decisions might not be what we would choose, or what we think is best. However, when we can show the patient that they can trust us, that we will support them and continue to contribute toward their health and well-being, they may well begin to make thoughtful movement toward wellness.

Each dimension can be approached in this format:

- Spiritual
- Cultural
- Social
- Emotional

We can ask "What matters to you?" of each patient to start the dialogue. From the simplest preference, like wanting to have their bath in the evening instead of the morning, to the more complex understanding of the impact of family and cultural dynamics on their overall healthcare; understanding the person will allow us to give them the best possible care. A goal all healthcare professionals share.

We want to know: "What do I need to know about you as a person, to give you the best possible care?"

CHAPTER 9

Conclusion

Nurses are compassionate people, and we want to help others – we're altruistic. Yet, it can be difficult to help others when our actions aren't appreciated by some of our patients. We may have grown up in a culture where holding a person's hand and making eye contact communicated our caring. Taking over with the solution to the person's problem, telling them not to worry, and giving them instructions for what to do is a prevailing mind-set for how to provide care.

But in a pluralistic society, we might feel shocked or insulted when our efforts to provide compassionate care are rebuffed or are considered offensive. We may have learned about different cultures in school or in-service education; even considering ourselves culturally competent. Yet, the truth is that all cultures are internally diverse, and generalities are not going to help much when working with individuals.

We also work with a variety of people in our organizations. We often feel the sting of not being treated with respect by those organizations, and are frustrated with the healthcare system – a system that seems too huge to be able to change. We might hear about the importance of self-care; resilience, taking yoga classes, having "me time," and many more tools. Those things can certainly be helpful, and we should do the things that serve us. We cannot, though, fix the healthcare system by taking a yoga class.

What we can do, and what we owe ourselves, is have compassion for ourselves. Only you can know what the best course is for yourself if you're feeling burned-out, or experiencing empathic distress, or even moral injury. It could be that you need a change, and there are many avenues in healthcare that you can pursue. Nurses have many skills that are valuable in other fields as well.

You might want to stay in your current role, and be willing to take on some steps to make things better on your unit. If you are a nurse leader, you can look for ways to be the best leader you can be. It's often said, and studies show, that staff don't leave the organization, they leave their manager. We've all worked for toxic managers, yet if we asked those managers why they do the things they do, they may well feel that they have no choice; that the system is dictating how they manage.

Can you turn things around? Realistically, you will have to manage under the constraints of the system. There are things you can do to make your unit's environment far more acceptable to work in. By asking you staff "What matters to you?" listening to the answers, and doing what you can to follow up on making things better, you'll go a long way toward returning the pride and even joy in work. When people are proud of the work they are doing, they go home tired for sure, but proud to make a difference.

By centering compassion in everything we do, we don't treat anyone as expendable or merely a means to an end. Each person on the healthcare team is a valuable member deserving of compassion, respect, and dignity. The patients we serve are not just room numbers and disease processes. They have full lives that include many priorities that might not center on their medical condition.

In all of this, using the C.A.R.E. process will clarify and simplify what to do in any given situation. In Compassion Centered C.A.R.E., we see the whole person and, while we might not always agree with their decisions, we can accept their choices as right for them in that moment. Compassion also gives us hope that when the person feels that we respect them, wish the best for them, and are doing our best to help them, that they can trust us. They might even decide that we've earned their trust, and may be more willing to try our advice, especially when it's crafted to fit with their lifestyle and values.

What's Next?

If you are a front line nurse leader, it's important that you know your situation:

- ✓ Are your staff's patient plans of care individualized?
- ✓ Does your staff understand their patient's social determinants of health?
- ✓ Are the patient's priorities and preferences respected and part of the plan of care and discharge plan?

Knowing where the knowledge gaps are will help in your efforts for education and training. Many times staff will complain about individualized plans of care, considering them "too hard," or not understanding how the plan can be individualized. They wonder, "Aren't all gall bladder surgeries the same?" not realizing that the differences in response to a surgery, treatment, or medication is only a small part of what makes the plan specific to the patient.

Staff may need additional education and training about the social determinants of health. Learning about how the systemic, social, and socioeconomic factors impact their patients helps staff know what questions to ask, and understanding that it's really not the patient's fault that they have difficulties following the discharge plan. They may be surprised to know that the lifestyle advice we love to give our patients might not have nearly the impact we wish they had.

But most important in this framework is the understanding of the patient's priorities and preferences. The patient is a partner in care, and compliance isn't necessarily the ultimate goal, while developing trust, treating the patient with respect, and honoring their culture and world view definitely is. The discharge plan is a crucial part of patient care. Only when we look at our patients as the team leader of their care, and see the big picture of their life will we be able to create a plan that will be successful and bring about the outcomes we hope for.

When we put this framework into action, we will see improvements in our care. Use these assessment prompts to evaluate:

- ✓ Seeing the patient as a person and a partner in care
- ✓ Improved individualized plans of care and discharge planning
- ✓ Improved patient satisfaction, reduced readmission rates, and improved compliance

Celebrate your success! Your patients will feel respected, will make better choices, and have improved outcomes.

Bibliography

Agency for Healthcare Research and Quality. (2018). CAHPS Clinician and Group Survey Measures. Rockville, MD. http://www.ahrq.gov/cahps/surveys-guidance/cg/about/survey-measures.html

Barnes-Neff, Cheryl. (2021). CARE: Connect, Assess, Respond, Evaluate. *CLOSLER Lifelong Learning in Clinical Excellence*. https://closler.org/lifelong-learning-in-clinical-excellence/3-priorities-in-palliative-care

Baughan, J. and Smith, A. (2013). *Compassion, Caring, and Communication*. New York, NY: Routledge, Taylor Francis Group.

Brown, Brené. (2013) Brené Brown on Empathy. *The RSA Org*. https://youtu.be/1Evwgu369Jw

Dignity in Care. (2016). Dignity in Care Toolkit. http://www.dignityincare.ca/en/toolkit.html

Dudgeon, K. (2015). Understanding the Whole Patient: A Model for Holistic Care. *Continuum Innovation.* Retrieved online on 4/28/2019: https://www.continuuminnovation.com/en/how-we-think/blog/understanding-the-whole-patient/

Erickson, M., Sandor, K. (Revised 2017). Core Essentials for the Practice of Holistic Nursing *The American Holistic Nurses Credentialing Corporation*.

Fogarty, RX. (2020). #DearNurses. *Dear World.org*.

https://nurses.dearworld.org/013-I-ve-Never-Cried-Like-That-About-A-Patient-1

Grassman, Deborah. (2019). Anchoring Heart Technique. *Opus Peace Soul Inquiry*. https://opuspeace.org/soul-injury-inventory/soul-restoring-resources/anchoring-heart/

Guo, Q., et al. (2017). Development and Evaluation of the Dignity Talk Question Framework for Palliative Patients and Their Families. *Palliative Medicine*, Vol. 32(1) 195-205.

Halifax, Joan. (2018). *Standing at the Edge: Finding Wisdom Where Fear and Courage Meet.* New York, NY: Flatiron Books.

Institute for Healthcare Improvement. (2019). What Matters Information Page. Retrieved online on 4/29/2019: http://www.ihi.org/Topics/WhatMatters/Pages/default.aspx

Lee, Thomas. (2016). *An Epidemic of Empathy in Healthcare: How to Deliver Compassionate, Connected Patient Care That Creates a Competitive Advantage*. New York, NY: McGraw-Hill Education.

Luxford, K. (2015). Rising to the Challenge of Patient-Centered Care. *Health Management: The Journal*. Volume 15, Issue 3.

Mapping Therapy Goals to the International Classification of Functioning, Disability, and Health. (2019). *Centers for Medicare and Medicaid Services*. Retrieved online on 4/29/2019: https://www.cms.gov/Medicare/Billing/TherapyServices/Downloads/Mapping_Therapy_Goals_ICF.pdf

Ozcan, T. (2018). Can We Evaluate and Treat the Patient as a Whole? *Health Management: The Journal*. Volume 18, Issue 6. 448-450.

Perlo J, Balik B, Swensen S, Kabcenell A, Landsman J, Feeley D. (2017). IHI Framework for Improving Joy in Work: IHI White Paper. *Institute for Healthcare Improvement*. http://www.ihi.org/resources/Pages/IHIWhitePapers/Framework-Improving-Joy-in-Work.aspx

Price, R.A. et al. (2018). Development of Valid and Reliable Measures of Patient and Family Experiences of Hospice Care for Public Reporting. *Journal of Palliative Medicine*, Volume XX, Number XX.

Prodinger, B., Rastall, P., Wooldridge, D., & Carpenter, I. (2018). Documenting Routinely What Matters to People: Standardized Headings for Health Records of Patients with Chronic Health Conditions. *Applied Clinical Informatics*. Volume 9, No. 2/2018.

Rogers, Fred. (2018). Mr. Rogers' Neighborhood. https://www.misterrogers.org/

Seppälä, Emma. (2020). Social Connection Boosts Health, Even When You're Isolated, Social connection is Key to Health and Happiness. *Psychology Today.* https://www.psychologytoday.com/us/blog/feeling-it/202003/social-connection-boosts-health-even-when-youre-isolated

Trzeciak, S. and Mazzarelli, A. (2019). *Compassionomics: The Revolutionary Scientific Evidence That Caring Makes a Difference.* Pensacola, FL: Studer Group Publishing.

Weisman, Theresa. (1996). A Concept Analysis of Empathy. *Journal of Advanced Nursing*. 23, 1162-1167.

What is a Holistic Health Assessment? (2019). Lamar University, Beaumont, TX. Retrieved online on: 4/29/2019: https://degree.lamar.edu/articles/nursing/holistic-health-assessment.aspx

World Health Organization. International Classification of Functioning, Disability, and Health. Information page, updated 2 March 2018. Retrieved on 4/29/2019: https://www.who.int/classifications/icf/en/

Zamanzadeh, V, Jasemi, M, Valizadeh, L, Koegh, B., & Taleghani, F. (2015). Effective Factors in Providing Holistic Care: A Qualitative Study. *Indian Journal of Palliative Care*. 21(2). 214-224.

Acknowledgements

There are many people to acknowledge and thank. I want to thank my editor, and the wonderful people at Laurel Oak Press for their help and support. There have been many mentors along the way, and I'd like to thank Sylvia Parker my nurse mentor when I began working in hospice for helping me understand a more holistic way to see my patients, Carmen Demos and Jillian Madsen for honing my work on the holistic conceptual framework, and the many nurses who listened to my talks and classes, and gave me invaluable feedback and encouragement.

I would also like to acknowledge and thank my family. My son Chris and partner Matt have been such a strong support throughout this adventure in creating courses and this book. Even though they have had to put up with my late nights, helping me through frustrations with the computer, and listening to me go on and on about some new idea or concept, they were always there for me.

Lastly, I must thank my bestie and mother-in-law, Carol Foster without whom this book would not exist. Through her own adventures in writing, I have learned a lot about editing, book publishing, book design – we have learned together, and I look forward to more fun with books!

About the Author

Cheryl Barnes-Neff has been a Registered Nurse for over forty years, with decades of management and quality improvement experience. Having worked in a variety of healthcare settings from neonatal intensive care to hospice care, she developed an understanding for the importance of quality nursing care. With a commitment to lifelong learning, she has earned a number of certifications, two Master's degrees, and a Doctorate.

Always interested in culture and religion, she has immersing herself in both through learning and travel. This interest has enabled her to integrate patient care in not only the physical, but the psychosocial, spiritual, and cultural dimensions. She found her calling in hospice care, and has spent over twenty years as a hospice nurse, educator, quality manager, and chaplain.

During her career, she's seen many patient care models come and go: From team nursing, to primary care, to care management, all the way to today's most popular model, patient centered care. None of those models takes a holistic view of healthcare, and her proposal is that our care model should actually be Compassion Centered C.A.R.E. With compassion in the center, we're applying compassion to ourselves, our co-workers, and to our patients and their families.

For More Information

For more information about Compassion Centered C.A.R.E., please visit ***barnesneff.com*** to read additional articles about compassion, care, and nursing leadership.

Continuing education courses are available, including free one hour credit courses on the *Introduction to Compassion Centered C.A.R.E.* and *Holistic Assessment*. An in depth workshop *C.A.R.E. About What Matters* is also available to take a deeper dive into how to apply these important concepts.

Enroll in our learning portal to find out more, and sign up for classes at:
https://courses.barnesneff.com/

Connect with me on Social Media at:

LinkedIn

https://www.linkedin.com/in/cheryl-barnes-neff/

Instagram

https://www.instagram.com/cheryl.barnes_neff/

Twitter

https://twitter.com/BarnesNeff

Facebook

https://www.facebook.com/authorcherylbarnesneff

NOTES

NOTES

NOTES

NOTES

Made in United States
North Haven, CT
29 April 2026

10630503R00062